Understanding Trichotillomania

A Path to Hair Pulling Disorder Recovery

Dr Mukesh Aggarwal

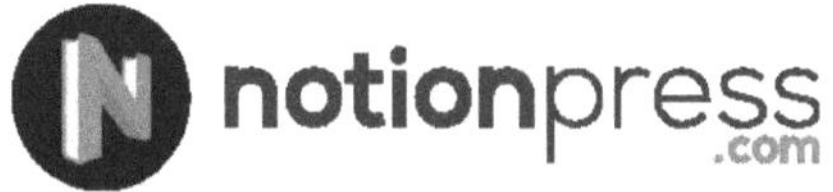

CONTENTS

PREFACE

In the fabric of human experience, there exists a spectrum of challenges that test our resilience and understanding. Trichotillomania, a subtle yet profound disorder, traverses this spectrum, often shrouded in misconceptions and overlooked intricacies. As a clinician, I have witnessed the enigmatic nature of this condition and the profound impact it has on those it touches.

This book, 'Understanding Trichotillomania: A Path to Hair Pulling Disorder Recovery', is an endeavor born from a passion to demystify and alleviate the burdens of this complex disorder. It stands as a testament to the amalgamation of clinical insights, personal stories, and the unwavering pursuit of a clearer path to recovery.

Through these pages, I am not only to provide knowledge but also to offer solace, guidance, and a compassionate hand in traversing the multifaceted landscapes of trichotillomania. May this book serve as a source of understanding, resilience, and hope for all those touched by this intricate condition.

With Gratitude
Dr Mukesh Aggarwal

UNVEILING TRICHOTILLOMANIA

Trichotillomania is a mental health condition characterized by an irresistible urge to pull out hair, leading to noticeable hair loss. It's often a way to cope with stress or anxiety. Therapy, support groups, and sometimes medication can help manage it. If you or someone you know is dealing with this, seeking professional help is important for understanding and addressing it effectively.

Definition and Diagnosis of Trichotillomania

Trichotillomania, a psychological disorder falling under the category of body-focused repetitive behaviors (BFRBs), involves the recurrent pulling out of one's hair, leading to hair loss and significant distress or impairment in social, occupational, or other important areas of functioning. This condition manifests differently in individuals, but the primary characteristic is the irresistible urge to pull out hair from the scalp, eyebrows, eyelashes, or other body areas, resulting in noticeable hair loss.

The diagnosis of trichotillomania involves certain criteria set forth by the Diagnostic and Statistical Manual of

Mental Disorders (DSM-5). To be diagnosed, an individual must exhibit recurrent hair pulling, resulting in hair loss, repeated attempts to decrease or stop hair pulling, and significant distress or impairment in various areas of life due to the behavior. Furthermore, the symptoms should not be better explained by another mental or medical condition.

Assessment for trichotillomania involves a comprehensive evaluation by a mental health professional, typically a psychologist or psychiatrist. This evaluation includes a thorough clinical interview to gather information about the individual's symptoms, history, and any contributing factors or coexisting conditions. It may also involve self-report measures, observations, and collaboration with other healthcare providers to rule out any underlying medical causes.

Differentiating trichotillomania from other conditions, such as dermatological disorders or other psychiatric conditions involving hair loss, is crucial in the diagnostic process. Professionals often consider the duration, severity, and impact of the behavior on the individual's life when making a diagnosis.

Treatment for trichotillomania commonly involves a combination of approaches, including cognitive-behavioral therapy (CBT), habit reversal training, acceptance and commitment therapy (ACT), and sometimes medication. CBT aims to identify triggers and develop coping strategies to manage the urge to pull hair, while habit reversal techniques focus on replacing the pulling behavior with alternative actions. Medications such as selective serotonin reuptake inhibitors (SSRIs) may be prescribed in some cases to help manage symptoms.

In conclusion, trichotillomania is a complex psychiatric disorder characterized by recurrent hair pulling resulting in noticeable hair loss, distress, and impairment. Its diagnosis requires careful evaluation by mental health professionals to differentiate it from other conditions and create an effective treatment plan tailored to the individual's needs. Early recognition and intervention are essential for improving outcomes and enhancing the individual's quality of life.

Symptoms of trichotillomania and variations across individuals

Trichotillomania manifests differently across individuals, but some common symptoms include:

Hair pulling: An irresistible urge to pull hair from the scalp, eyebrows, eyelashes, or other body areas.

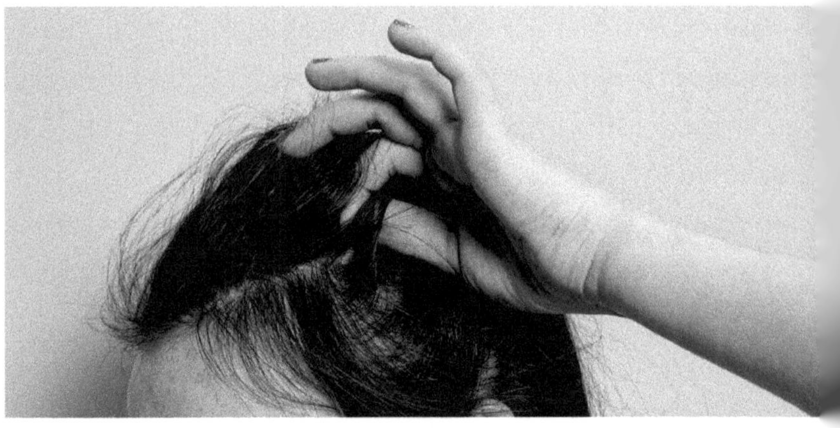

Tension before pulling: Feeling increasing tension or anxiety before pulling out hair.

Sense of relief or gratification: A feeling of relief, pleasure, or satisfaction after pulling out hair.

Attempts to stop: Repeated unsuccessful attempts to decrease or stop hair pulling.

Distress or impairment: Significant distress or impairment in social, occupational, or other important areas of functioning due to the behavior.

Noticeable hair loss: Patchy bald spots or thinning hair in affected areas.

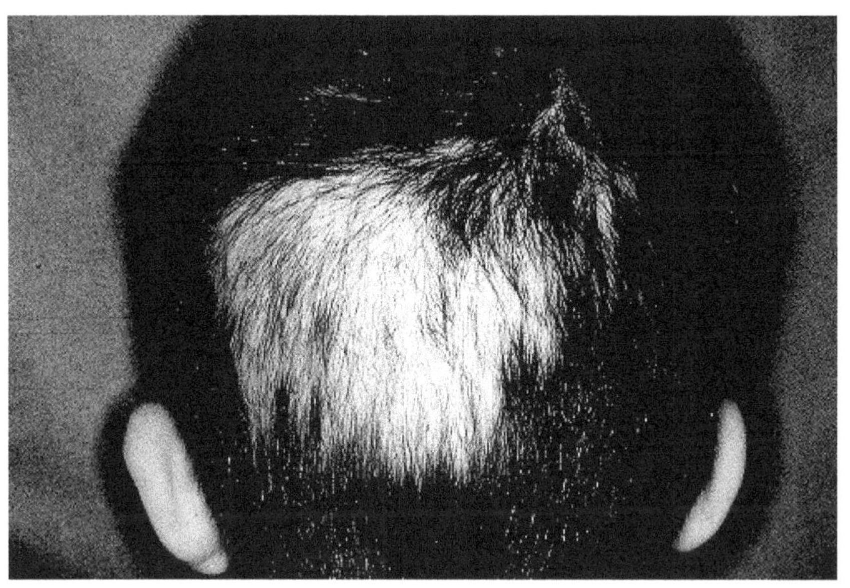

Variations in symptoms can include the frequency and severity of hair pulling, the areas targeted for hair removal, and the emotional and psychological impact on individuals. Some may engage in the behavior consciously, while others may do so involuntarily or habitually without awareness.

Triggers for hair pulling and the emotional context surrounding the behavior can also vary widely among individuals. Understanding these variations is crucial in tailoring effective treatment approaches for each person dealing with trichotillomania.

Prevalence and demographics of trichotillomania

Trichotillomania, though considered a relatively rare condition, affects individuals across diverse demographics. Its prevalence rates vary across studies, with estimates suggesting a prevalence of approximately 0.5% to 2% in the general population. However, due to underreporting and the private nature of the disorder, the actual prevalence might be higher than reported.

This disorder often begins in childhood or adolescence, with symptoms typically surfacing between the ages of 9 and 13. However, it can emerge at any age. Females are more commonly affected than males, with many studies indicating a female-to-male ratio of around 3:1 or higher.

The disorder's impact on various demographic groups is an area of ongoing research. Still, studies suggest that trichotillomania can affect individuals from diverse cultural, socioeconomic, and ethnic backgrounds. However, societal and cultural factors may influence the expression and reporting of symptoms, potentially impacting prevalence rates across different communities.

In terms of comorbidities, individuals with trichotillomania often experience other mental health conditions, such as anxiety disorders (particularly obsessive-compulsive disorder), depression, or various impulse control disorders. Understanding these associations is crucial in providing comprehensive care and effective treatment strategies for individuals dealing with trichotillomania.

Additionally, trichotillomania can have a significant impact on individuals' quality of life, leading to social withdrawal, academic or occupational impairment, and difficulties in relationships. Seeking professional help is essential for accurate diagnosis, appropriate intervention, and support for affected individuals.

Research into the prevalence and demographics of trichotillomania continues to evolve, aiming to better understand its incidence across different populations, improve diagnostic methods, and develop more targeted interventions to address this complex disorder.

TRIGGERS AND CAUSES

Triggers can vary widely, often linked to stress, anxiety, boredom, or even certain situations or emotions. Causes aren't fully understood, but genetics, brain chemistry, and environmental factors likely play a role.

Psychological and emotional triggers of Trichotillomania

Trichotillomania's psychological and emotional triggers encompass a complex interplay of factors. Stress, a prevalent trigger, often exacerbates the condition, leading to increased hair pulling episodes. Anxiety, whether related to specific situations or generalized, can intensify the urge to pull hair as a coping mechanism.

Emotional distress, such as feelings of frustration, loneliness, or low self-esteem, commonly coexist with trichotillomania. Individuals may resort to hair pulling as a means of seeking relief or regaining a sense of control amidst emotional turmoil.

Boredom acts as another trigger, with idle moments or lack of stimulation prompting subconscious hair-pulling behaviors. Moreover, negative emotional states like guilt or shame arising from the act of pulling itself can perpetuate a distressing cycle, fostering further episodes.

The psychological root causes of trichotillomania often intertwine with underlying mental health conditions like anxiety disorders, obsessive-compulsive disorder (OCD), or depression. Additionally, trauma or adverse childhood experiences might contribute to its onset or exacerbation.

Understanding and addressing these psychological and emotional triggers through therapy, particularly cognitive behavioral therapy (CBT), can empower individuals with strategies to manage impulses, regulate emotions, and break the cycle of hair pulling. Support groups and mindfulness practices also play a pivotal role in fostering awareness and providing coping mechanisms for individuals dealing with trichotillomania.

Genetic predispositions and neurological factors of Trichotillomania

Trichotillomania's connection to genetic predispositions and neurological factors underscores the intricate nature of this impulse control disorder. Studies suggest a hereditary component, indicating a higher likelihood of developing trichotillomania if a close family member also experiences the condition.

Genetic predispositions manifest in variations within specific genes associated with brain development, neurotransmitter regulation, and impulse control mechanisms. Variants in genes related to the serotonin system, which influences mood and behavior, have been implicated in some cases of trichotillomania. This suggests a potential link between neurotransmitter imbalances and the disorder's onset.

Neurologically, trichotillomania involves alterations in brain structures and functions. Imaging studies have highlighted differences in brain activity and connectivity, particularly in regions associated with impulse control, such as the prefrontal cortex. These findings suggest that neurological differences might contribute to the difficulty in regulating the urge to pull hair.

Moreover, dysregulation in neurotransmitters like serotonin, dopamine, and glutamate, which modulate mood, reward, and inhibitory control, could play a significant role in the development and perpetuation of trichotillomania. These neurotransmitter imbalances may affect the brain's reward system, influencing the reinforcing nature of hair pulling behavior.

While genetic predispositions and neurological factors offer insights into the underpinnings of trichotillomania, they likely interact with environmental influences and psychological stressors. This intricate interplay highlights the multifaceted nature of the disorder, requiring a holistic approach to treatment.

Therapeutic interventions, including cognitive behavioral therapy (CBT), aimed at modifying behaviors and addressing underlying emotional triggers, coupled with medication targeting neurotransmitter imbalances, form the basis of effective management strategies. Research into the genetic and neurological aspects of trichotillomania continues, holding promise for more targeted and personalized treatments in the future.

Environmental influences on trichotillomania

Environmental influences wield a substantial impact on the manifestation and progression of trichotillomania, intersecting with genetic predispositions and psychological triggers. These influences encompass a wide array of external factors that contribute to the development or exacerbation of this complex impulse control disorder.

Early life experiences and upbringing constitute influential environmental factors. Adverse childhood events, trauma, neglect, or stressful environments may serve as precipitating elements in the onset of trichotillomania. Such experiences can mold coping mechanisms, potentially leading to maladaptive behaviors like hair pulling as a means of managing distress.

Family dynamics and learned behaviors within the household also influence trichotillomania. Observing or experiencing certain behaviors related to stress management or emotional regulation within the family context might impact an individual's propensity to resort to hair pulling as a coping mechanism.

Social factors, including peer pressure, social stigma, or bullying, can exacerbate emotional distress, triggering or intensifying episodes of hair pulling. Additionally, societal beauty standards and the pressure to conform to certain appearances might heighten feelings of self-consciousness or anxiety, contributing to the compulsion to pull hair.

Stressful life events, major transitions, or ongoing difficulties in various life domains, such as academic, professional, or personal spheres, can act as precipitating factors or exacerbate existing symptoms of trichotillomania. High-stress situations often intensify the urge to pull hair, serving as catalysts for hair-pulling episodes.

Furthermore, access to tools or environments conducive to hair pulling, such as tweezers or periods of isolation, can facilitate and reinforce the behavior.

Recognizing and addressing these environmental influences is crucial in the comprehensive treatment of trichotillomania. Therapeutic interventions, including cognitive behavioral therapy (CBT) and family therapy, aim to identify and mitigate these environmental stressors while equipping individuals with coping mechanisms to manage triggers effectively.

Creating supportive environments, promoting resilience, and fostering understanding and acceptance within social circles and communities play pivotal roles in the successful management and recovery from trichotillomania. An integrated approach that acknowledges both genetic predispositions and environmental influences is key to effective treatment strategies for this challenging disorder.

Chapter 3

THE EMOTIONAL LANDSCAPE

Trichotillomania can create a complex emotional landscape. Individuals often feel a range of emotions like shame, guilt, frustration, and anxiety due to the compulsive urge to pull out their hair. They might also experience relief or satisfaction temporarily after pulling, followed by regret or distress. Seeking professional support is crucial to manage these emotions and address the condition effectively.

Impact on self-esteem and confidence

The impact of trichotillomania on self-esteem and confidence can be profound. The compulsive urge to pull out hair often leads to visible patches or bald spots, triggering feelings of embarrassment, shame, and self-consciousness.

For many, the inability to control this behavior can severely diminish self-esteem. The constant worry about others noticing the hair loss can lead to social withdrawal and avoidance of situations where their condition might be exposed. This further undermines confidence in social interactions and professional settings.

Moreover, the cycle of pulling, feeling relief or satisfaction temporarily, and then experiencing regret and distress can create an emotional rollercoaster. This fluctuation can erode one's self-image, leading to a negative perception of oneself.

Over time, the emotional toll of trichotillomania can result in a significant reduction in self-worth and confidence. However, seeking support from mental health professionals, support groups, and therapies tailored for trichotillomania can help individuals manage their condition, regain self-esteem, and rebuild confidence. With understanding, support, and appropriate interventions, it's possible to address the emotional impact of trichotillomania and foster a more positive self-image.

Relationships and social interactions

Trichotillomania, while primarily affecting an individual's relationship with themselves, can significantly influence their interactions within social circles and relationships.

Impact on Relationships:

Social Withdrawal: Trichotillomania often leads to self-consciousness about visible hair loss, prompting individuals to withdraw from social situations. This withdrawal can strain friendships and limit the formation of new connections.

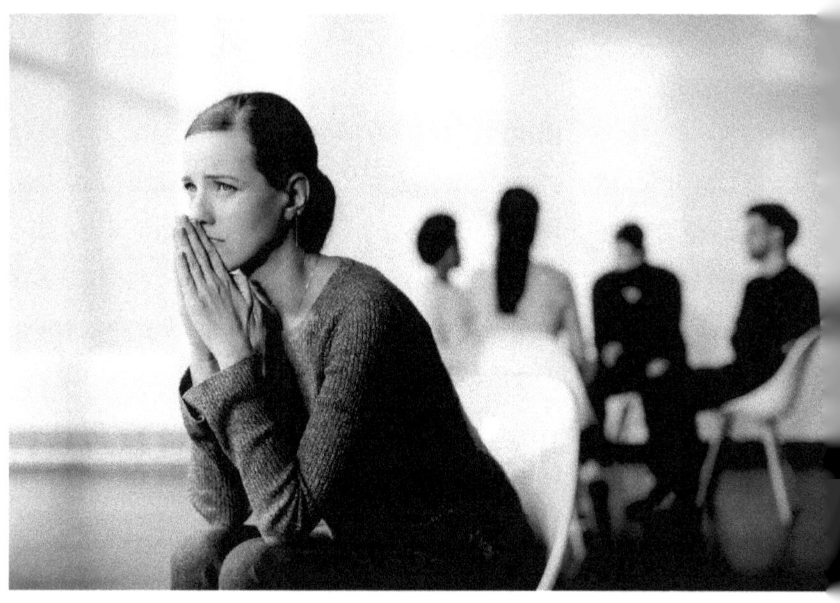

Difficulty Explaining the Condition: Many individuals with trichotillomania find it challenging to explain their condition to others, fearing judgment or misunderstanding. This communication barrier might hinder intimacy and trust within relationships.

Impact on Intimacy: In romantic relationships, the secrecy or shame associated with trichotillomania can affect intimacy and openness. Fear of rejection or embarrassment may hinder individuals from disclosing their condition, leading to strained relationships.

Social Interactions:

Stigma and Misunderstanding: Societal misconceptions about hair pulling disorders can lead to stigmatization. This misunderstanding might cause discomfort or isolation in social settings, impacting the individual's ability to engage comfortably.

Performance in Social Situations: The anxiety and distress caused by trichotillomania can affect an individual's performance in social situations. Fear of judgment or embarrassment might hinder their ability to fully participate in social activities or conversations.

Impact on Confidence: Trichotillomania's effect on self-esteem can directly impact how individuals present themselves socially. Lower self-confidence might make them appear reserved, impacting their ability to form new relationships or maintain existing ones.

Addressing trichotillomania's impact on relationships and social interactions often involves a combination of therapy, support groups, and open communication. Encouraging understanding and empathy within social circles can create a supportive environment, enabling individuals to feel accepted and understood despite their condition. Building awareness about trichotillomania in society can also help reduce stigma, fostering an inclusive environment for those affected.

Coping mechanisms and emotional management for a person having trichotillomania

Coping Mechanisms and Emotional Management for Trichotillomania

Trichotillomania, characterized by the compulsive urge to pull out hair, often requires multifaceted approaches for coping and emotional management.

1. Awareness and Mindfulness: Understanding triggers and recognizing the urge to pull hair are crucial. Mindfulness techniques, like deep breathing or grounding exercises, can help individuals pause and redirect their attention when experiencing the urge.

2. Behavioral Therapy: Cognitive Behavioral Therapy (CBT) tailored for trichotillomania can assist in identifying and altering negative thought patterns and behaviors associated with hair pulling. This therapy helps individuals develop healthier coping strategies.

3. Habit Reversal Training (HRT): HRT aims to replace hair-pulling behaviors with alternative actions. This technique involves awareness training, learning competing responses (like clenching fists instead of pulling), and receiving social support.

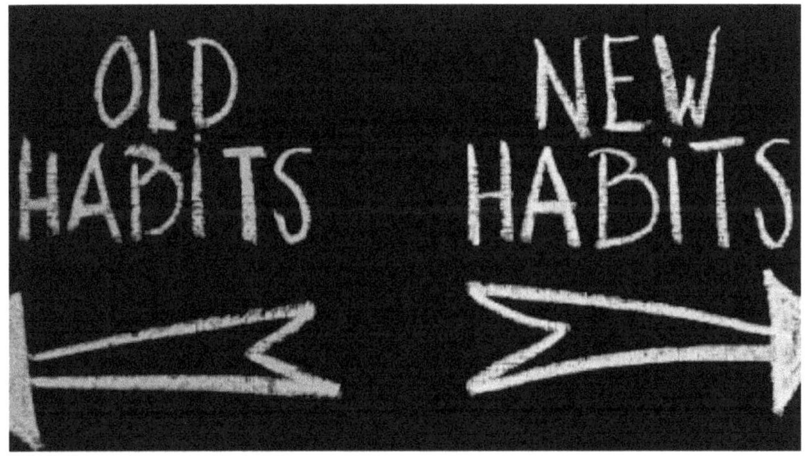

4. Stress Management: Stress often exacerbates trichotillomania. Engaging in stress-relieving activities such as exercise, meditation, or hobbies can reduce the intensity of the urge to pull.

5. Support Groups and Therapy: Joining support groups or undergoing individual therapy provides a safe space for sharing experiences and gaining support. Peer encouragement and professional guidance aid in developing effective coping mechanisms.

6. Environment Modification: Making changes to the environment can reduce the likelihood of hair pulling. For instance, wearing hats or gloves, keeping hands occupied with stress balls, or rearranging spaces to minimize access to hair can be helpful.

7. Self-Care and Positive Reinforcement: Encouraging self-care practices, such as maintaining a healthy lifestyle, adequate sleep, and practicing self-compassion, can positively impact emotional well-being and reduce triggers.

8. Medication and Professional Help: In severe cases, medication, prescribed by healthcare professionals, might be considered to manage associated anxiety or depression.

Combining these strategies based on individual needs and preferences is vital for effectively managing trichotillomania. It's essential to approach treatment holistically, addressing both the behavioral and emotional aspects of the condition. Seeking professional guidance ensures tailored interventions, empowering individuals to cope better and manage their emotional responses effectively.

TREATMENT OF TRICHOTILLOMANIA

Treating trichotillomania often involves a combination of therapy, medications, and alternative approaches. Therapy options include Cognitive Behavioral Therapy (CBT), Habit Reversal Training (HRT), and Acceptance and Commitment Therapy (ACT). Medications like SSRIs or NAC can also aid in managing symptoms. Alternative approaches encompass mindfulness, support groups, and relaxation techniques. These treatments aim to reduce pulling behaviors, address underlying triggers, and enhance coping mechanisms for individuals with trichotillomania.

Medical treatment of trichotillomania

The medical treatment of trichotillomania primarily involves the use of medications and supplements to manage symptoms and aid in controlling the compulsive hair-pulling behavior. Selective Serotonin Reuptake Inhibitors (SSRIs), such as fluoxetine (Prozac), fluvoxamine (Luvox), and sertraline (Zoloft), have shown effectiveness in reducing the urges and symptoms associated with trichotillomania.

N-Acetylcysteine (NAC), a supplement that affects glutamate levels in the brain, has also demonstrated promise in some studies for reducing hair-pulling symptoms. It's believed to modulate the neurotransmitter systems involved in compulsive behaviors, though individual responses may vary.

The effectiveness of medications can differ from person to person, and it might take some time to find the most suitable option and dosage. Regular monitoring by a healthcare professional is essential to assess progress and adjust treatments as needed.

Combining medication with therapy, particularly Cognitive Behavioral Therapy (CBT) or Habit Reversal Training (HRT), tends to yield better outcomes. These therapies help individuals identify triggers, develop coping strategies, and modify the behavior associated with trichotillomania.

It's important to note that while medications can be beneficial, they might not entirely eliminate the urge to pull hair. Therefore, a holistic approach that combines medication with therapy and other supportive measures is often recommended for effective management of trichotillomania. Regular communication with healthcare providers ensures comprehensive and personalized care for individuals dealing with this condition.

Alternative treatment for trichotillomania

Alternative treatments for trichotillomania encompass various approaches beyond conventional medication and therapy. These approaches aim to complement traditional treatments and offer additional avenues for managing symptoms and reducing hair-pulling behaviors.

Mindfulness and Meditation: Practices like mindfulness-based techniques and meditation can help individuals increase self-awareness, manage stress, and develop better impulse control. Mindfulness encourages being present in the moment, which can assist in recognizing and interrupting the urge to pull hair.

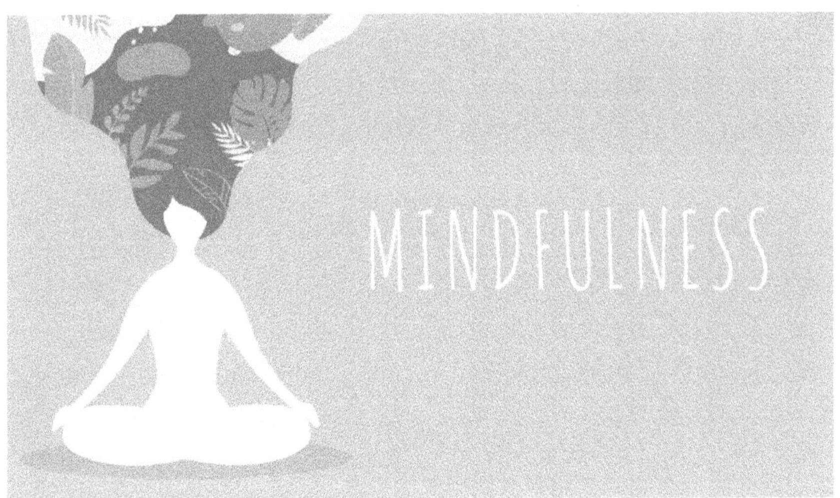

Yoga and Exercise: Engaging in physical activities like yoga or exercise routines can reduce stress and anxiety, which are often triggers for trichotillomania. Regular exercise helps regulate mood and can contribute to better overall mental health.

Aromatherapy and Essential Oils: Some people find relief from symptoms through the use of aromatherapy or essential oils known for their calming effects. Scents like lavender, chamomile, or bergamot may help promote relaxation and reduce anxiety, potentially alleviating the urge to pull hair.

Acupuncture: While research is limited, acupuncture, a traditional Chinese practice involving the insertion of thin needles into specific points of the body, is sometimes explored as a complementary therapy. It's believed to rebalance energy flow and may aid in reducing stress and anxiety associated with trichotillomania.

Support Groups and Peer Support: Connecting with others who share similar experiences through support groups or online communities can provide a sense of belonging, understanding, and encouragement. Sharing experiences and coping strategies with peers can be invaluable in managing trichotillomania.

Biofeedback and Habit Reversal Devices: Biofeedback techniques and habit reversal devices can help individuals become more aware of their pulling behaviors. These methods involve using technology to track and alert individuals when they engage in hair-pulling, aiding in self-awareness and behavior modification.

It's important to note that the effectiveness of alternative treatments can vary from person to person, and these methods might not work as standalone solutions. Combining alternative approaches with evidence-based therapies under the guidance of healthcare professionals often yields the most comprehensive and effective outcomes for managing trichotillomania. Consulting with a healthcare provider before starting any alternative treatment is recommended to ensure safety and suitability for individual needs.

Challenges In Seeking Help For Trichotillomania

Stigma and Shame: There's often a stigma attached to compulsive behaviors, causing individuals to feel embarrassed or ashamed about their condition. This can prevent them from seeking help or disclosing their struggles.

Lack of Awareness: Trichotillomania isn't as widely understood as some other mental health conditions, leading to misconceptions and a lack of awareness among the general public and sometimes even healthcare professionals.

Difficulty in Diagnosis: Trichotillomania might be misdiagnosed or overlooked due to similarities with other conditions. Some individuals might not recognize their symptoms as a diagnosable disorder, delaying or inhibiting their decision to seek help.

Limited Access to Specialists: Accessing mental health professionals or specialists well-versed in treating trichotillomania can be challenging, especially in areas with limited mental health resources.

Treatment Effectiveness and Persistence: Finding an effective treatment might take time, and some individuals might feel discouraged if initial treatments don't yield immediate results. Consistency and persistence in treatment are crucial but can be challenging.

Financial Barriers: Costs associated with therapy, counseling, or medications might hinder access to treatment, especially if individuals don't have adequate insurance coverage or financial resources.

Overcoming these challenges often requires patience, perseverance, and a supportive environment. Increased awareness, destigmatization efforts, and accessible mental health services can significantly aid individuals in seeking and receiving the necessary help and support for managing trichotillomania.

Support System And Resources Available For Trichotillomania

Creating a robust support system is crucial for individuals dealing with trichotillomania. Several resources and supportive networks are available to provide assistance, guidance, and a sense of community for those affected by this condition.

Support Groups: Joining local or online support groups specifically dedicated to trichotillomania allows individuals to connect with others facing similar challenges. Sharing experiences, coping mechanisms, and successes within these communities fosters a sense of understanding and reduces feelings of isolation.

Non-Profit Organizations and Advocacy Groups: Various non-profit organizations, such as the Trichotillomania Learning Center (TLC) and the Canadian BFRB Support Network, offer valuable resources, information, and support for individuals, families, and caregivers affected by trichotillomania and related disorders.

Therapy and Counseling: Seeking professional help from therapists or counselors specializing in trichotillomania can provide personalized strategies to manage symptoms. Cognitive Behavioral Therapy (CBT) and Habit Reversal Training (HRT) are commonly recommended therapeutic approaches.

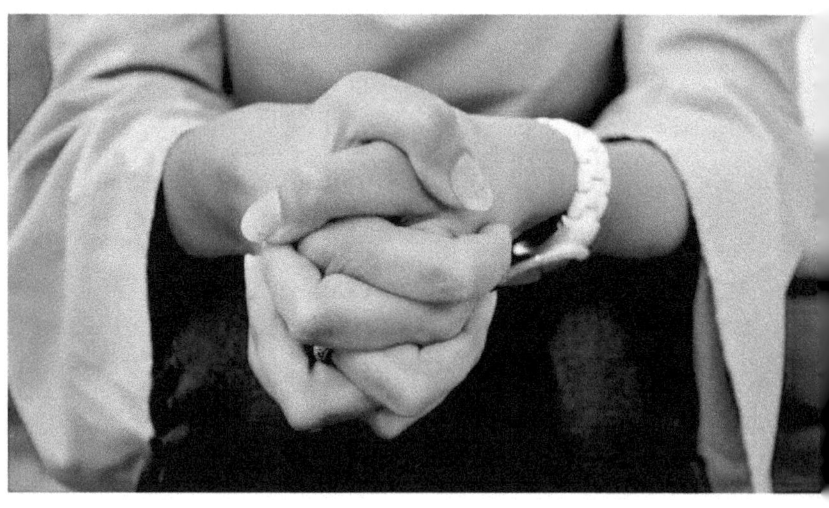

Online Forums and Communities: Online forums, social media groups, and community platforms provide accessible spaces where individuals can seek advice, share stories, and access resources anonymously. Websites like Reddit'sr / Trichsters or dedicated Facebook groups facilitate discussions and support for those with trichotillomania.

Educational Materials and Websites: Reliable online resources and educational materials provided by reputable sources like the TLC website, Mayo Clinic, or the Anxiety and Depression Association of America offer comprehensive information about trichotillomania, treatment options, coping strategies, and tips for managing symptoms.

Hotlines and Helplines: Some organizations or mental health services offer hotlines or helplines where individuals can seek immediate support, guidance, or crisis intervention related to trichotillomania or other mental health concerns.

Building a support system involves tapping into a combination of these resources. The support system can include friends, family members, healthcare providers, and online or in-person communities. Each element contributes to a network of understanding, empathy, and guidance, aiding individuals in navigating the challenges of trichotillomania and fostering a sense of empowerment and hope.

STORIES OF TRIUMPH

Many individuals have found success through a combination of therapy, support groups, self-awareness techniques, and personal determination. Some have shared their journeys online through blogs, vlogs, or social media, highlighting their progress and offering support to others facing similar challenges. It's a testament to the human spirit's resilience and the power of perseverance in overcoming such difficulties.

Success Stories And Experiences Of Overcoming Trichotillomania

Story 1: One inspiring story is that of a woman who battled trichotillomania for years. Through therapy, she developed coping mechanisms such as wearing gloves or styling her hair differently to reduce the urge to pull. With support from family and friends, she gradually regained control.

Story 2: Another person found relief through a combination of cognitive behavioral therapy (CBT) and habit reversal training, learning to identify triggers and redirect the urge to pull.

Story 3: One remarkable success story involves a young woman named Sarah. She struggled with trichotillomania for over a decade, causing noticeable hair loss and immense emotional distress. Sarah reached a turning point when she decided to seek professional help. She started therapy sessions focusing on cognitive behavioral techniques specifically tailored to address her triggers and urges to pull.

Her therapist guided her through various exercises, teaching her to recognize the thoughts and emotions that triggered her pulling behavior. Sarah learned alternative behaviors to replace pulling, such as squeezing a stress ball or engaging in deep breathing exercises whenever she felt the urge. She also began using tools like fidget toys to keep her hands occupied.

Additionally, Sarah joined a support group where she found encouragement and understanding from others facing similar challenges. Sharing experiences and strategies with the group members made her feel less alone in her journey.

It wasn't an easy road, and setbacks occurred, but Sarah persisted. Over time, her dedication to therapy, the support of her group, and her commitment to the techniques she'd learned started showing results. The frequency of her pulling decreased significantly, and she noticed gradual hair regrowth.

With consistent practice and perseverance, Sarah regained control over her urges. She learned to manage stress more effectively and found healthier ways to cope. While the journey wasn't without its difficulties, Sarah's determination, combined with professional guidance and peer support, led her to a place of triumph over trichotillomania. Today, she proudly shares her story to inspire others and offer hope to those battling similar challenges.

These success stories showcase the power of therapy, support systems, and personal resilience in overcoming trichotillomania.

Insights and advice from individuals who have made progress

These are insights and advice shared by individuals who've made progress in managing their trichotillomania:

Identifying Triggers: Many have emphasized the importance of recognizing triggers that lead to pulling. Insights include understanding emotional states, specific situations, or thoughts that precede the urge to pull. Once identified, individuals can work on managing or avoiding these triggers.

Therapy and Professional Help: Seeking professional guidance, especially through cognitive behavioral therapy (CBT), has been instrumental for many. Learning coping strategies, relaxation techniques, and habit reversal training provided the tools needed to combat the urge to pull.

Support Systems: Building a support network has been crucial. Engaging with support groups or finding understanding friends and family members has helped individuals feel less isolated and more empowered in their journey toward recovery.

Alternative Coping Mechanisms: Developing alternative behaviors to replace pulling has been effective. Strategies like using fidget toys, stress balls, or keeping hands busy with activities such as drawing, knitting, or playing musical instruments have helped redirect the urge to pull.

Self-Care and Stress Management: Prioritizing self-care and stress reduction techniques has been emphasized. Exercise, mindfulness practices, relaxation exercises, and maintaining a healthy lifestyle have helped individuals better manage stress, reducing the urge to engage in hair pulling.

Patience and Persistence: Progress often takes time. Many advise being patient and kind to oneself throughout the journey, acknowledging that setbacks can happen but staying committed to the recovery process is key.

These insights and advice collectively highlight the multifaceted approach to managing trichotillomania, emphasizing the importance of professional guidance, support, self-awareness, and persistence in achieving progress and control over the condition.

Understanding And Supporting Loved Ones With Trichotillomania

Trichotillomania is a mental health condition characterized by the compulsive urge to pull out one's hair. When a loved one is grappling with this disorder, the support and understanding of friends, family, and partners become invaluable. Here are some ways these close relationships can provide effective support:

1. Educate Yourself: Understanding trichotillomania is the first step toward offering meaningful support. Educate yourself about the condition, its triggers, and the challenges it presents. This knowledge will help you comprehend what your loved one is going through.

2. Encourage Professional Help: Gently encourages your loved one to seek professional assistance. Therapists, counselors, or psychologists specializing in trichotillomania can offer strategies and support tailored to their needs.

3. Practice Empathy and Patience: Be patient and empathetic. Trichotillomania is complex, and recovery takes time. Offer a non-judgmental, compassionate ear and avoid criticizing or making them feel ashamed of their behavior.

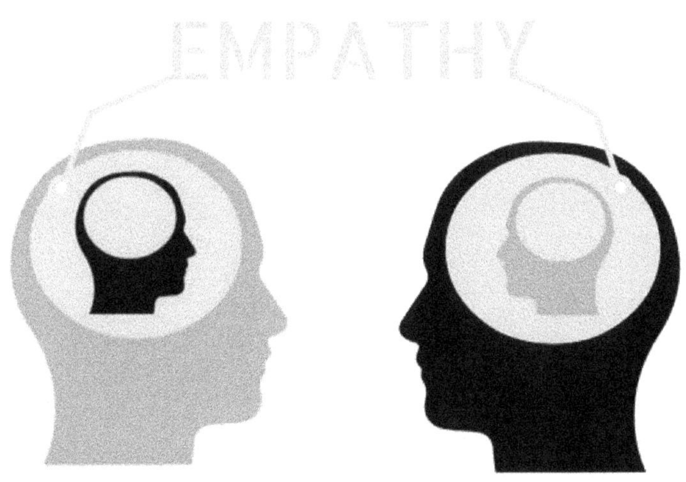

4. Engage in Open Communication: Encourage open communication without pressure. Let your loved one know that they can confide in you without fear of judgment. Be available to listen whenever they are ready to share.

5. Help Identify Triggers and Coping Mechanisms: Assist your loved one in identifying triggers that exacerbate their pulling behavior. Together, explore healthy coping mechanisms and alternative behaviors that can redirect the urge to pull.

6. Be Supportive in Treatment Plans: If your loved one is undergoing treatment, offer your support. Attend therapy sessions if invited, participate in activities that promote relaxation and stress reduction, and assist in implementing strategies learned in therapy.

7. Foster a Positive Environment: Create a positive and supportive environment. Celebrate small victories and progress made in managing the condition. Encourage self-care practices that promote overall well-being.

8. Join Support Groups: Encourage participation in support groups or communities where individuals dealing with trichotillomania can share experiences, strategies, and encouragement. Knowing they're not alone can be immensely comforting.

9. Take Care of Yourself: Supporting someone with trichotillomania can be emotionally taxing. Remember to take care of your own well-being, seek support from others, and set boundaries to maintain your own mental health.

In conclusion, supporting a loved one with trichotillomania requires patience, empathy, and understanding. By educating oneself, fostering open communication, and encouraging professional help, friends, family, and partners can play a crucial role in aiding their loved one's journey toward recovery. Creating a supportive and non-judgmental environment is key to helping them feel understood, accepted, and empowered to manage their condition.

MOVING FORWARD

Moving forward with trichotillomania can involve various strategies. Seeking professional help, such as therapy or counseling, can assist in managing and understanding the condition. Developing coping mechanisms, like keeping hands busy or using fidget toys, can also be beneficial. Additionally, exploring relaxation techniques or mindfulness practices might help in reducing the urge to pull hair. Remember, progress might take time, so be patient and kind to yourself along the way.

Long-Term Management And Relapse Prevention Of Trichotillomania

Managing trichotillomania over the long term involves a multifaceted approach that combines therapeutic interventions, lifestyle adjustments, and ongoing self-awareness. This condition, characterized by the recurrent urge to pull out one's hair, can significantly impact an individual's life, necessitating comprehensive strategies for management and relapse prevention.

Therapeutic Interventions: Therapy plays a pivotal role in long-term management. Cognitive-behavioral therapy

(CBT) has proven effective in treating trichotillomania. Through CBT, individuals learn to identify triggers and develop coping mechanisms to manage the urge to pull hair. Techniques such as habit reversal training, where individuals replace hair-pulling behaviors with alternative actions, contribute significantly to behavioral modification. Additionally, acceptance and commitment therapy (ACT) can help individuals acknowledge their urges without acting on them, fostering resilience against relapse.

Support Networks: Building a robust support network is instrumental in managing trichotillomania. Engaging with support groups or finding a supportive community can provide a sense of belonging and understanding. Sharing experiences, tips, and strategies within these groups can offer valuable insights and emotional support, reducing feelings of isolation and stigma often associated with this condition.

Lifestyle Adjustments: Adopting a holistic approach to health is crucial. Regular exercise, adequate sleep, and a balanced diet contribute to overall well-being, potentially reducing stress levels and the urge to pull hair. Incorporating stress-reduction techniques such as mindfulness, meditation, or yoga into daily routines can alleviate anxiety and manage triggers associated with trichotillomania.

Relapse Prevention: Maintaining vigilance against triggers is essential for preventing relapses. Continued therapy sessions or periodic check-ins with mental health professionals help individuals stay attuned to their emotional states and identify potential triggers. Developing a relapse prevention plan, which includes coping strategies and emergency contacts, empowers individuals to navigate challenging moments and prevent setbacks.

Acknowledging Setbacks: Despite efforts toward long-term management, setbacks may occur. It's imperative to approach these setbacks with self-compassion and without self-judgment. Seeking immediate support from professionals or the established support network can prevent a relapse from becoming a prolonged setback.

In conclusion, the long-term management of trichotillomania requires a comprehensive approach encompassing therapeutic interventions, lifestyle adjustments, support networks, and a proactive stance against potential relapses. By incorporating these strategies into daily life and staying committed to ongoing self-care, individuals affected by trichotillomania can work towards managing the condition effectively and enhancing their overall quality of life.

The Future of Trichotillomania

The future of trichotillomania treatment and research holds promise for improved understanding, innovative therapies, and increased awareness. Trichotillomania, a complex psychiatric disorder characterized by recurrent hair pulling, has garnered attention from researchers and clinicians striving to advance treatment approaches and deepen insights into its underlying mechanisms.

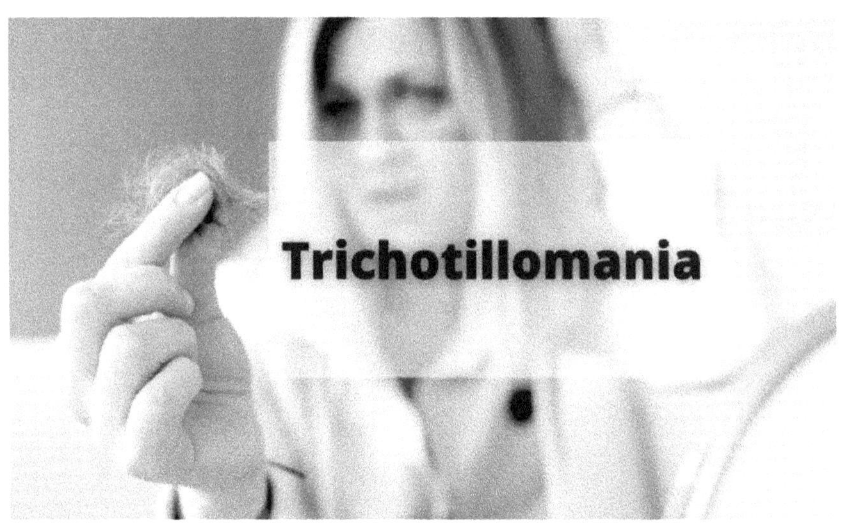

Advancements in Neurobiological Understanding: Emerging research focuses on the neurobiological underpinnings of trichotillomania. Exploring brain imaging techniques, such as functional MRI (fMRI) or PET scans, helps in identifying specific brain regions and neural pathways associated with the condition. These studies offer valuable insights into the neurocircuitry involved in impulse control, emotion regulation, and reward processing, potentially paving the way for targeted interventions.

Innovative Therapeutic Approaches: The landscape of therapeutic interventions for trichotillomania continues to evolve. Besides established treatments like cognitive-behavioral therapy (CBT) and habit reversal training (HRT), novel therapeutic modalities, including transcranial magnetic stimulation (TMS) or deep brain stimulation (DBS), are being explored. These techniques aim to modulate brain activity and disrupt maladaptive circuits implicated in trichotillomania, offering promising avenues for treatment.

Precision Medicine and Personalized Treatments: Advancements in genetics and personalized medicine hold potential for tailoring treatments to individuals with trichotillomania. Genetic studies seek to identify specific genes or genetic markers associated with the condition, paving the way for targeted therapies based on an individual's genetic profile. Personalized treatment plans may become more effective and efficient by considering genetic predispositions and biological markers.

Digital Health Solutions: The integration of digital health tools, such as smartphone applications or wearable devices, presents an opportunity to enhance trichotillomania management. These tools can offer real-time monitoring, provide behavioral interventions, track triggers, and deliver support remotely, augmenting traditional therapies and promoting consistent self-management.

Enhanced Public Awareness and Support: Increasing public awareness about trichotillomania remains crucial. Education initiatives, advocacy efforts, and destigmatization campaigns are essential to foster understanding and support for individuals affected by the condition. By reducing stigma, promoting acceptance, and encouraging early intervention, society can create a more supportive environment for those living with trichotillomania.

Collaborative Research and Multidisciplinary Approaches: Collaboration among researchers, clinicians, advocacy groups, and affected individuals is key to advancing trichotillomania research and treatment. Multidisciplinary approaches that integrate insights from neuroscience, psychology, genetics, and technology foster a comprehensive understanding and pave the way for innovative, holistic treatment strategies.

In conclusion, the future of trichotillomania treatment and research is promising, marked by advancements in neurobiology, innovative therapeutic approaches, personalized medicine, digital health solutions, increased public awareness, and collaborative efforts. These developments hold the potential to transform the landscape of trichotillomania management, offering hope for more effective treatments and improved quality of life for those affected by this challenging condition.